Asma Korbi

Urinary incontinence

AF307699

Asma Korbi

Urinary incontinence

ScienciaScripts

Imprint

Any brand names and product names mentioned in this book are subject to trademark, brand or patent protection and are trademarks or registered trademarks of their respective holders. The use of brand names, product names, common names, trade names, product descriptions etc. even without a particular marking in this work is in no way to be construed to mean that such names may be regarded as unrestricted in respect of trademark and brand protection legislation and could thus be used by anyone.

Cover image: www.ingimage.com

This book is a translation from the original published under ISBN 978-620-6-72442-1.

Publisher:
Sciencia Scripts
is a trademark of
Dodo Books Indian Ocean Ltd. and OmniScriptum S.R.L publishing group

120 High Road, East Finchley, London, N2 9ED, United Kingdom
Str. Armeneasca 28/1, office 1, Chisinau MD-2012, Republic of Moldova, Europe
Printed at: see last page
ISBN: 978-620-8-16291-7

INTRODUCTION

In an environment where fertility is high, maternal health is a particularly important public health concern. The prevalence of urinary incontinence associated with pregnancy in disadvantaged environments has not been sufficiently studied to date. Information on this subject is limited to epidemiological data from surveys carried out in developed countries, where prevalence estimates range from 6% to 29%. Pelvic floor muscle dysfunction may be associated with trauma to these muscles in women who have experienced prolonged and difficult labour and expulsion.

There is no reason to believe that the prevalence of incontinence after childbirth is lower in disadvantaged areas than in developed countries. Indeed, the less than ideal conditions of labour and birth and the limited access to healthcare services prevalent in disadvantaged environments may actually increase the risk of trauma to the pelvic floor muscles.

There are a number of interventions available to prevent and treat urinary incontinence, including medication, medical devices and surgery. However, strengthening the floor muscles (RMPP) - which involves exercising the muscles involved in the passage of urine (particularly the pelvic floor muscles) - could be the easiest intervention to implement in disadvantaged environments as it does not require specific equipment, additional healthcare infrastructure or other expensive resources.

Non-invasive, easy to learn and practicable almost anywhere and at any time, RMPP has been presented as an appropriate and acceptable intervention for pregnant women and women who have given birth and are likely to be breastfeeding. The midwife is a key contact for women during pregnancy, childbirth and the post-natal period. She is qualified to provide appropriate, clear and concise information on a number of topics, such as perineo-sphincter disorders and the need for perineal re-education sessions.

She is particularly well qualified to provide information to women, as she herself can carry out pelvic floor re-education. However, although attitudes have changed over the years, these subjects are still rarely discussed spontaneously by patients, and taboos persist.

MATERIALS AND METHOD

Two questionnaires were drawn up: the questionnaire for women and the questionnaire for men. This is a prospective study of women who gave birth at the AZIZA OTHEMENA Hospital, Obstetrics and Gynaecology Department, between 10 February 2014 and 10 March 2014.

Inclusion and exclusion criteria :

All women were included in the study:

Who had given birth by vaginal delivery or caesarean section during the study period. All women were excluded from the study:

Who have a urological pathology refusing to take part in the study

Data collection and entry:

Data was collected using questionnaires designed for women (Appendix 1). This tool was structured in several sections in relation to the objectives of the present study.

The modules consisted of :

Socio-demographic profile;

Marital status, family and profession; Previous history

The birth process

Urinary leakage after childbirth

Assessing knowledge of perineal rehabilitation and its benefits.

The women were contacted by telephone after one month's initial contact to complete the final part of the questionnaire.

Midwife questionnaire :

This is a study conducted among midwives at hospitals, plannings and dispensaries in the Tunis and Nabeul regions from 1 March 2018 to 20 March 2018. Data were collected using questionnaires developed for midwives (Appendix 2). The questionnaire is composed of several sections related to the study objective.

Ethical considerations

Participation in the study was voluntary; all those recruited were free to accept or refuse to participate in the study. The objectives and procedures of the study were clearly explained to the participants so that they could give free and informed consent. Each participant was reassured about the confidentiality of the information obtained during the study and the results. The questionnaires were anonymous; no names were requested.

The aim of our work :

The aim of our work is : to study the frequency of stress urinary incontinence in the post-partum period

Assess midwives' knowledge of how to manage this condition.

Statistical study :

We entered our data from the questionnaires into an Excel file. We compared the means using a chi^2 test with a significance level of 0.05.

RESULTS

Women's questionnaire results: 70 women who gave birth between 10 February 2014 and 10 March 2014.

I. Epidemiological studies :

1. Age

✓ Our series included 1% of women aged under 20, 53% of women aged between 20 and 30 and 46% of women aged over 30 (Figure 1).

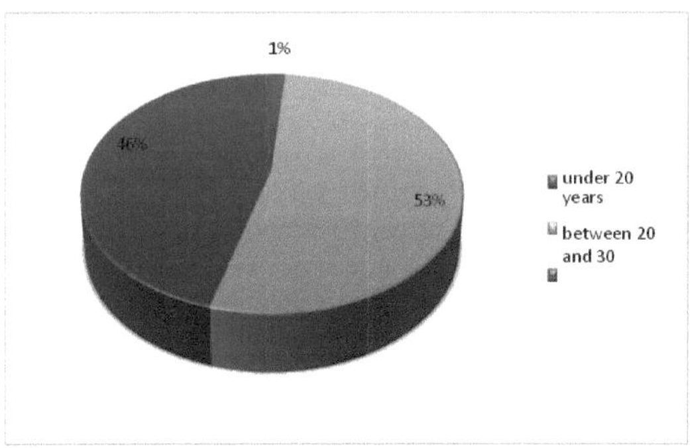

Figure 1: Age distribution.

2. Level of study

✓ The population studied is made up of 12% of illiterate women, 34% of women with primary education, 40% of women with secondary education and 14% of women with higher education (Figure 2).

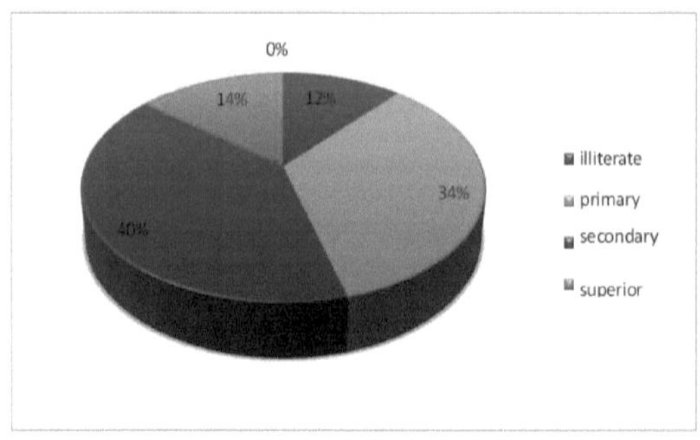

Figure 2: Breakdown by level of education.

3. Profession

✓ The majority of respondents to the questionnaire were housewives (Figure 3).

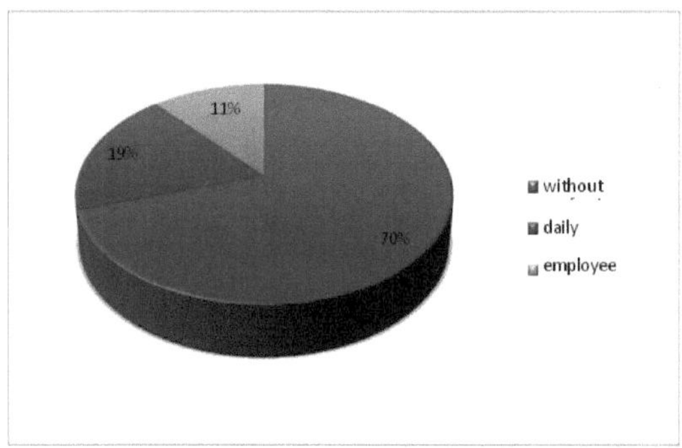

Figure 3: Breakdown by socio-professional category.

II. Background study

1. Parity

✓ 40% of the sample were primiparous women, 36% were 2nd pare women and

24% were 3rd pare women or more (figure 4).

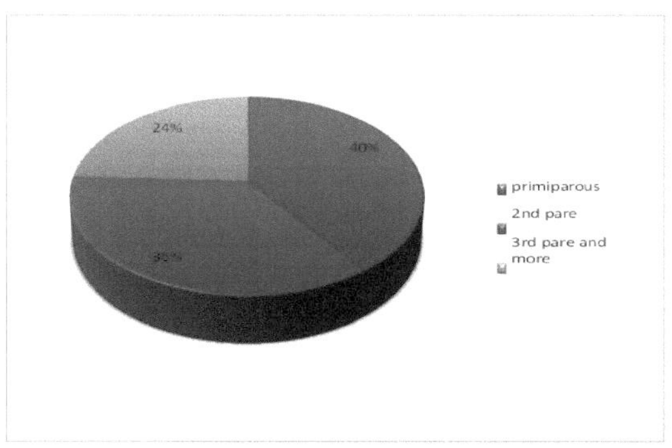

Figure 4: breakdown by parity.

2. Pregnancy

a. Weight gain during pregnancy :

✓ 56% of women stated that their weight gain during pregnancy was less than

10kg, 30% gained between 10 and 15kg and 14% gained more than 15kg

(Figure 5).

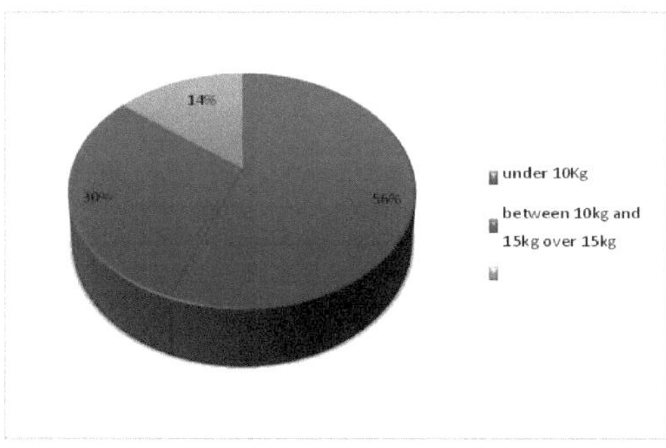

Figure 5: breakdown by weight gain.

b. Urinary leakage during pregnancy

√ 63% of women said they had experienced urine leakage during pregnancy, while 37% said they had not (Figure 6).

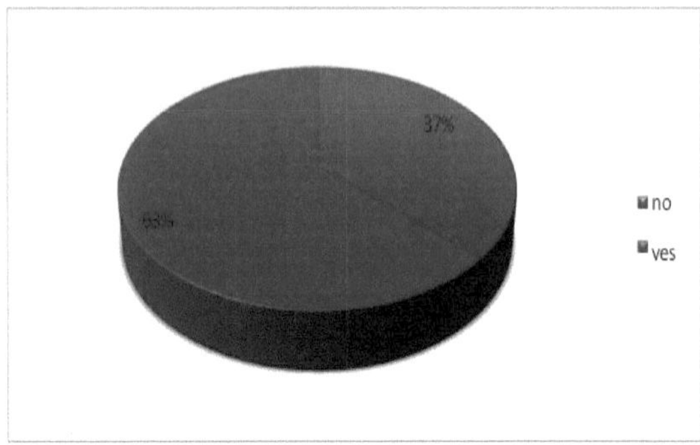

Figure 6: Urinary incontinence during pregnancy.

► If yes

√ Of the women who leaked urine during pregnancy, ½ leaked on coughing, ¼ leaked on physical exertion and ¼ leaked without physical exertion (Figure 7).

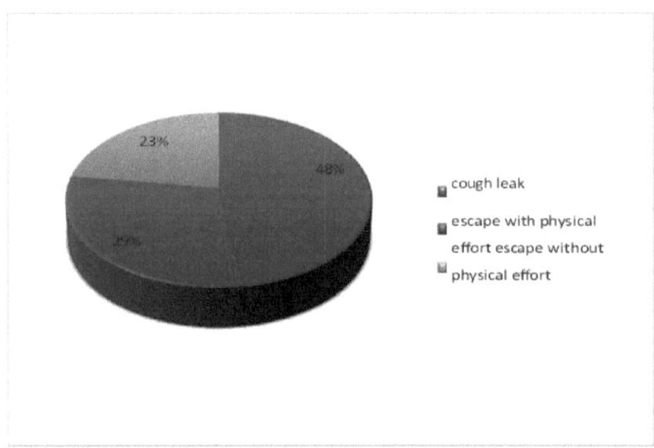

Figure 7: Types of urinary incontinence.

c. Birth preparation

✓ 17% of participants in the study had attended a birth preparation course, while

83% had never attended a birth preparation course (Figure 8).

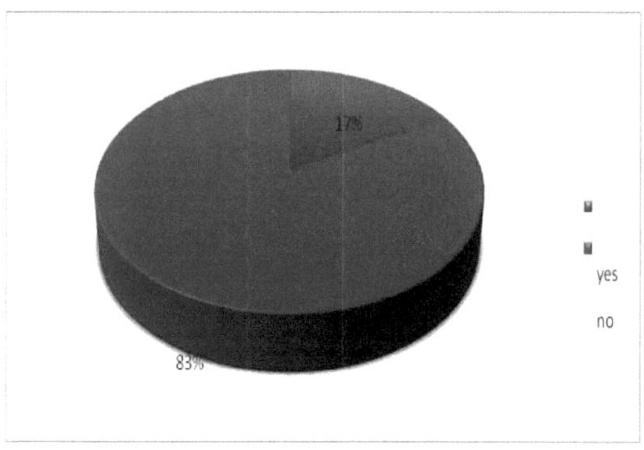

Figure 8: Birth preparation.

II.Giving birth

1. Term of delivery

✓ 7% of women gave birth before 37 weeks' gestation and 93% of women gave

birth at full term (Figure 9).

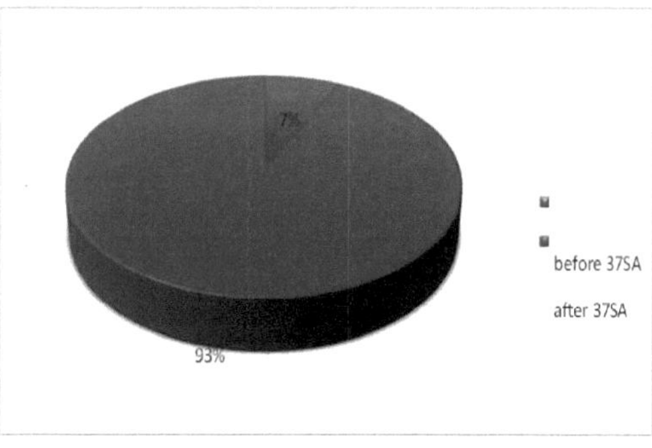

Figure 9: Breakdown by term of delivery.

2. Delivery method

√ 70% of deliveries were vaginal, of which 10% were assisted by forceps, and

30% were caesarean sections, of which 10% were scheduled and 20%

emergency (figure 10).

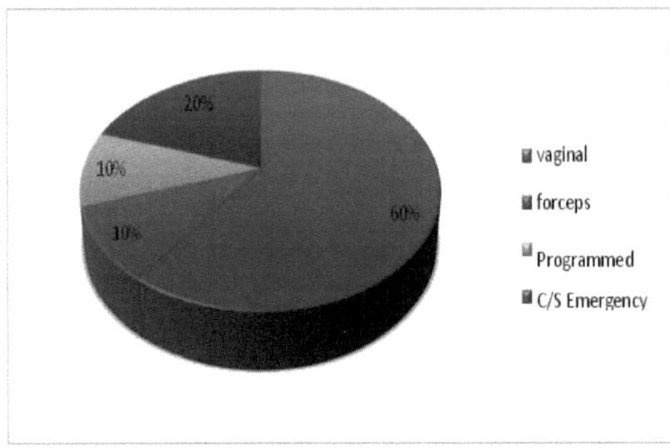

Figure 10: Breakdown by mode of delivery.

3. Evacuation bladder catheterisation :

√ In more than half of deliveries a bladder catheterisation was performed and

36% of deliveries were performed without a bladder catheterisation (Figure 11).

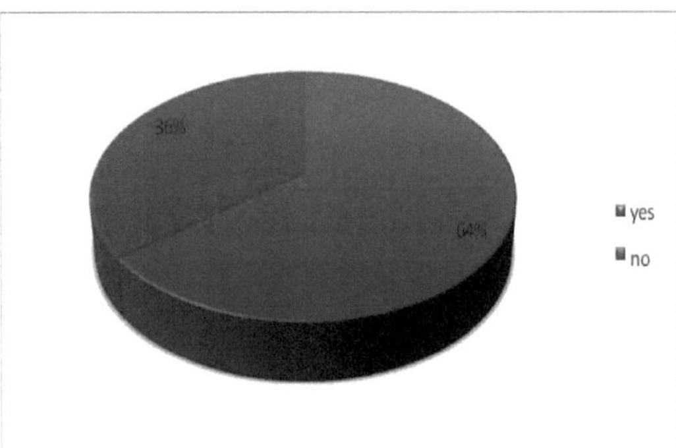

Figure 11: Use of bladder evacuation catheterisation.

4. Lesions of the perineum

✓   30% of patients had no injury to the perineum, 3% had a simple tear, no

patient had a complete tear and 67% had an episiotomy (Figure 12).

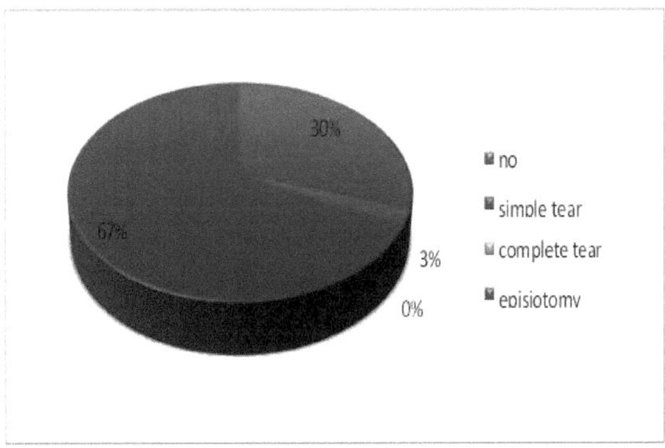

Figure 12: Distribution of lesions in the perineum.

5. Newborn weight

✓ Only 19% of newborns had a birth weight of over 3.7kg (Figure 13).

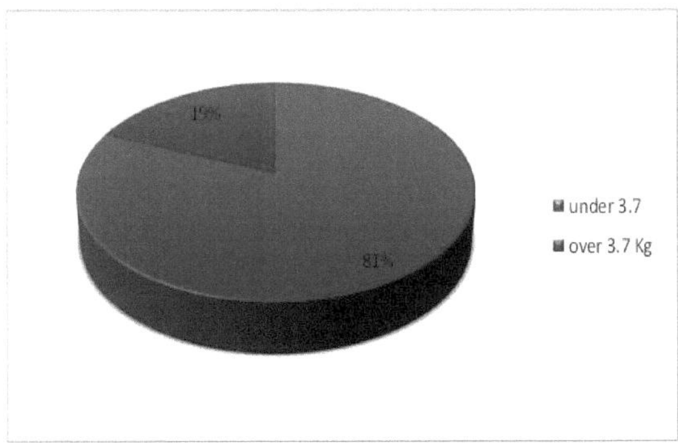

Figure 13: Breakdown by newborn weight.

6. Abdominal expression

√ In half of all vaginal deliveries, abdominal expression was performed (Figure 14).

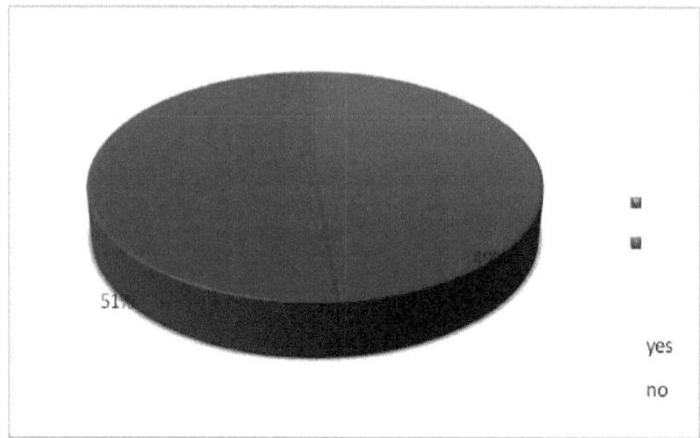

Figure 14: Distribution according to abdominal expression.

7. Knowledge of perineal rehabilitation

√ Only 11% of women had heard of perineal re-education, 4% of whom had heard of its benefits and 7% of patients who had heard of it but had no specific idea of its benefits (figure 15).

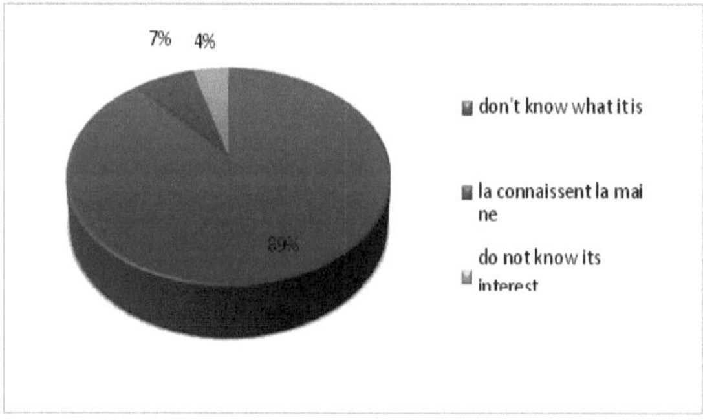

Figure 15: Distribution according to knowledge of perineal rehabilitation.

► Information resources

√ The only means of informing women about perineal reeducation has

was the media (figure16).

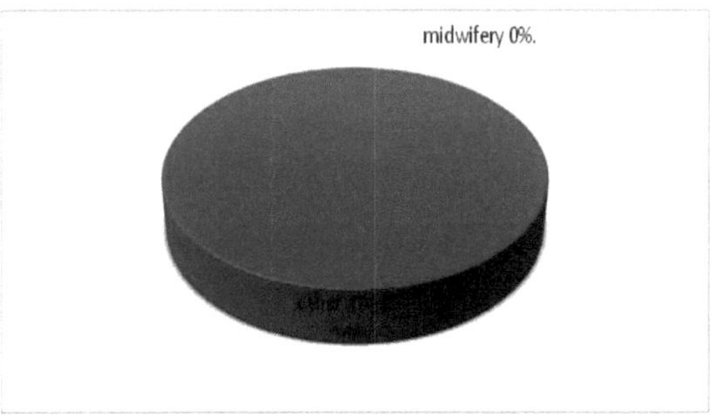

Figure 16: Information resources.

III. Results of 2ème part of the questionnaire:

1. Urinary leakage after one month's childbirth (post-partum)

√ After one month, only 19% of women experienced incontinence

urinary effort (figure17).

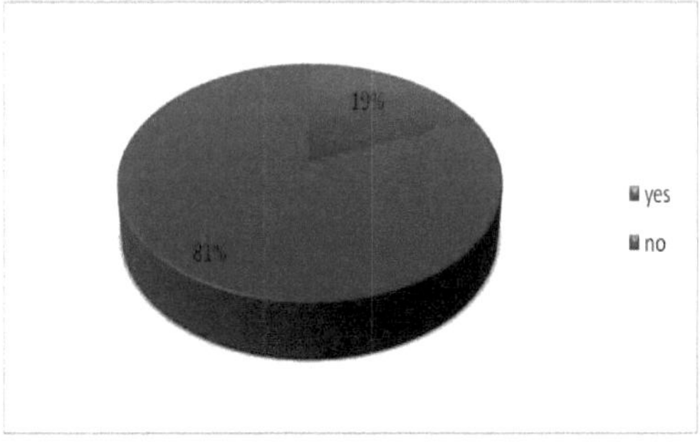

Figure 17: Reassessment of urinary incontinence 1 month after childbirth.

► If yes

✓   69% of women who reported postpartum urinary incontinence had cough-induced urine leakage, 16% had physical exertion-induced urine leakage and 15% had urine leakage without physical exertion (figure 18).

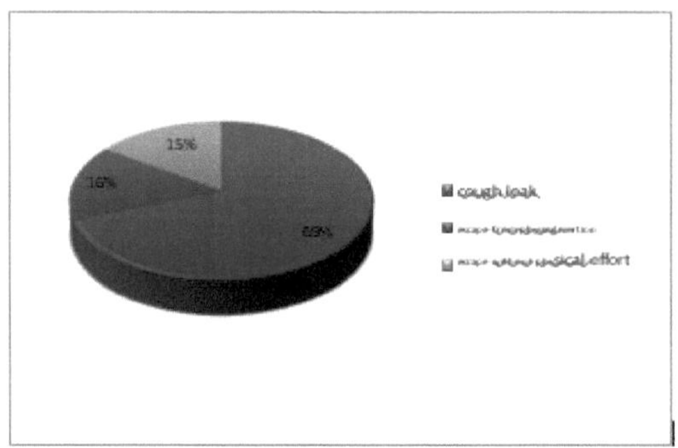

Figure 18: Type of urinary incontinence.

2. Planning to undergo perineal rehabilitation

► Healthy women

✓   7% of healthy women are expected to undergo perineal re-education (figure 19).

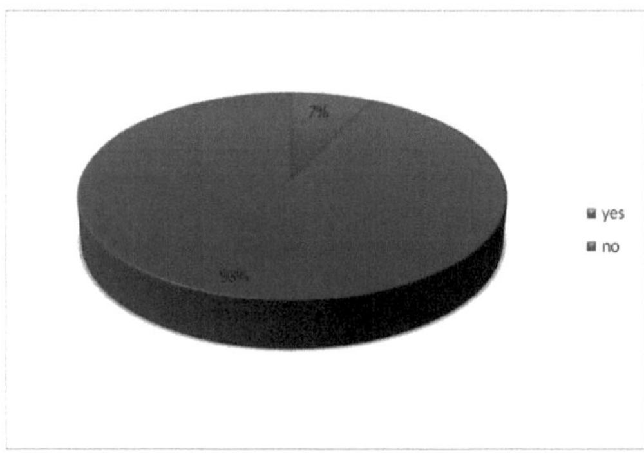

Figure 19: Plan to undergo perineal rehabilitation for healthy women.

► For the patients having a incontinence one month after childbirth

√ ½ of women who suffered from urinary incontinence post-partum wanted to undergo perineal re-education sessions (figure20).

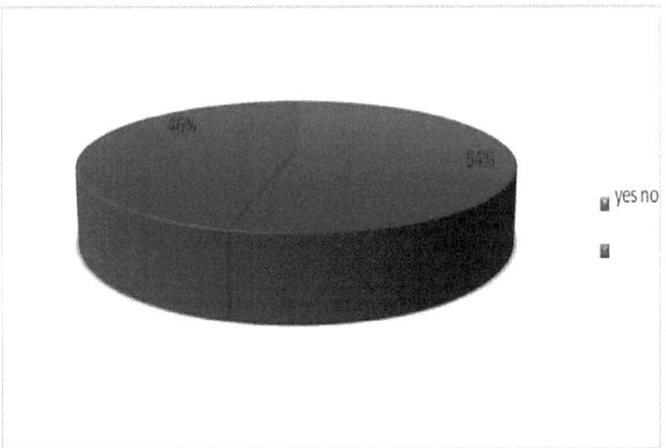

Figure 20: Plan to undergo perineal rehabilitation for incontinent women.

Results Midwife questionnaire: with 33 midwives at hospitals, plannings and dispensaries in the Tunis and Nabeul regions from 1ᵉʳ March 2014 to 20 March 2014.

I. Epidemiological studies :

1. Age :

√ Of the midwives surveyed, 9% were aged between 20 and 30, 23 were aged between 30 and 40, 24% were aged between 40 and 50 and 39% were aged over 50 (Figure 21).

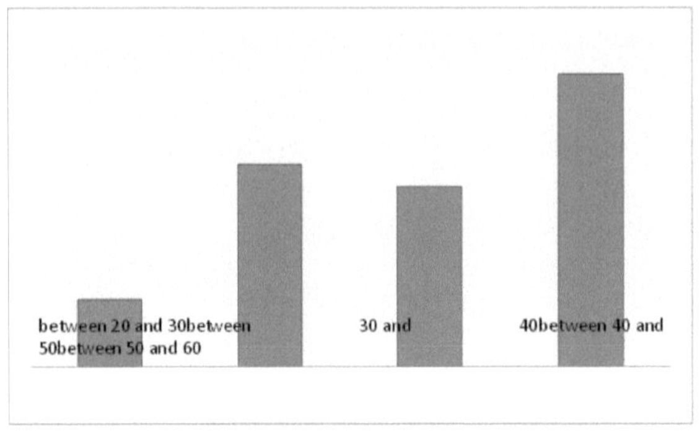

Figure 21: Age distribution of midwives.

2. Places of work :

The midwives who answered the questions worked in different positions (Figure 22).

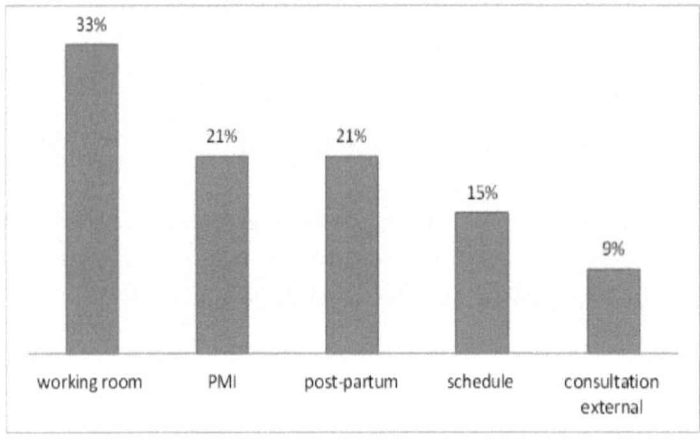

Figure 22: Breakdown by place of practice.

II. Knowledge about urinary incontinence :

1. Understanding urinary incontinence :

✓ 79% of midwives participating in the study had experienced postpartum urinary incontinence The midwives who answered the questions worked in different positions (Figure 23).

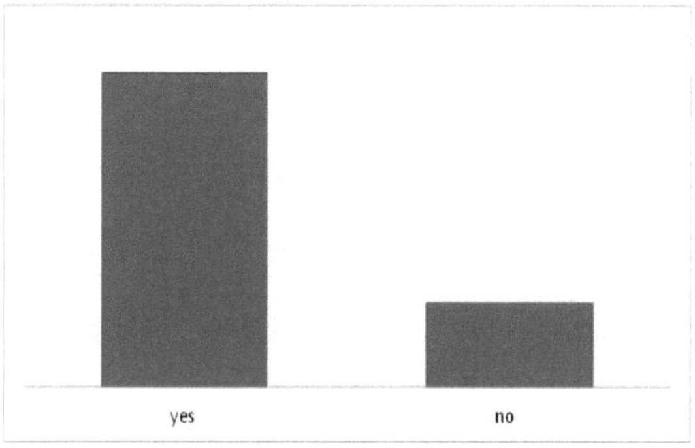

Figure 23: Distribution according to knowledge of urinary incontinence.

2. Knowledge of types of urinary incontinence:

✓ Only 46% of midwives knew the types of urinary incontinence The midwives who answered the questions work in different positions (Figure 24).

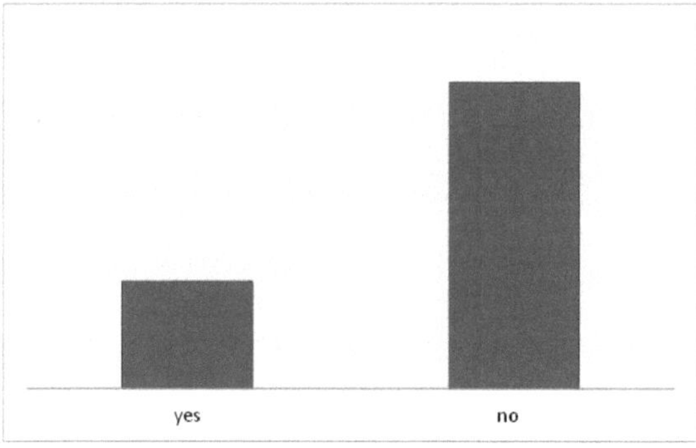

Figure 24: Distribution according to knowledge of types of incontinence.

3. Can you screen for post-partum urinary incontinence?

✓ 73% of midwives said they are able to screen for postpartum urinary

incontinence The midwives who answered the questions work in different

positions (Figure 25).

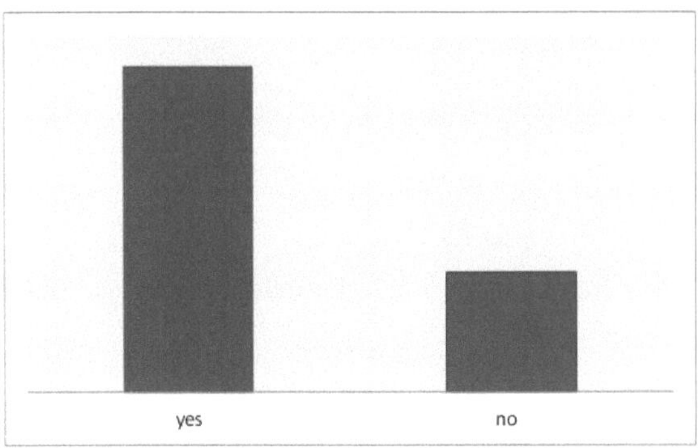

Figure 25: Urinary incontinence screening capacity.

4. How do we do it?

✓ In 84% of cases midwives used questioning as a means of screening, of which

5% carried out a clinical examination and in 11% used questioning and clinical

examination as a means of screening The midwives w h o answered the

questions worked in different positions (Figure 26).

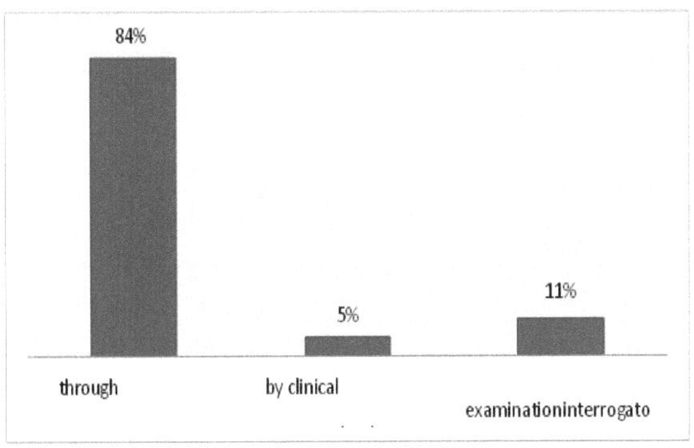

Figure 26: Screening methods.

5. Systematic screening :

✓ 42% of midwives have carried out systematic screening for urinary

incontinence The midwives who answered the questions work in different

positions (Figure 27).

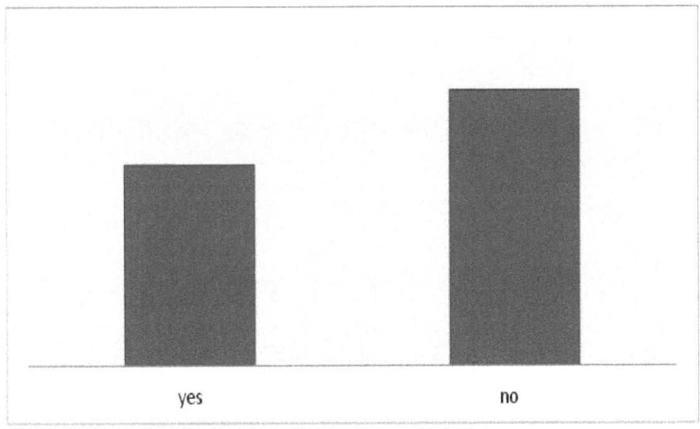

Figure 27: Systematic screening.

6. When is screening for post-partum urinary incontinence carried out?

✓   According to 15% of midwives, screening for urinary incontinence was done: during pregnancy ,21% early postpartum, 18% during the $8^{\text{ème}}$ day consultation ,9% during the $40^{\text{ème}}$ day consultation and 36% did not know when screening was done The midwives who answered the questions work in different positions (Figure 28).

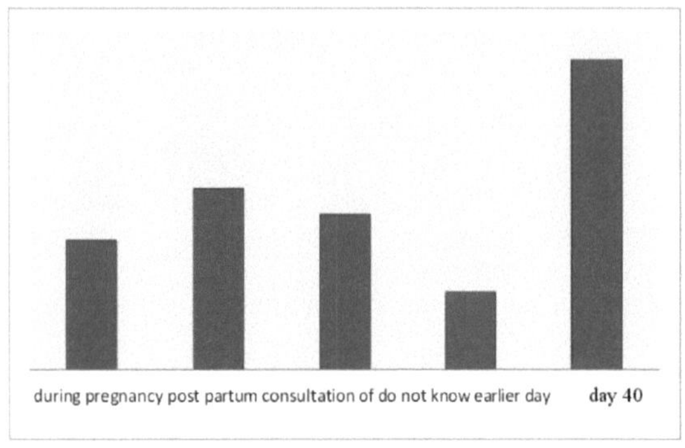

Figure 28: Date of incontinence screening.

7. Preventive measures for post-partum urinary incontinence :

✓ The most common preventive measure used by midwives was evacuation catheterisation during childbirth (55%) and preparation for childbirth (12%). The midwives who answered the questions work in different positions (Figure 29).

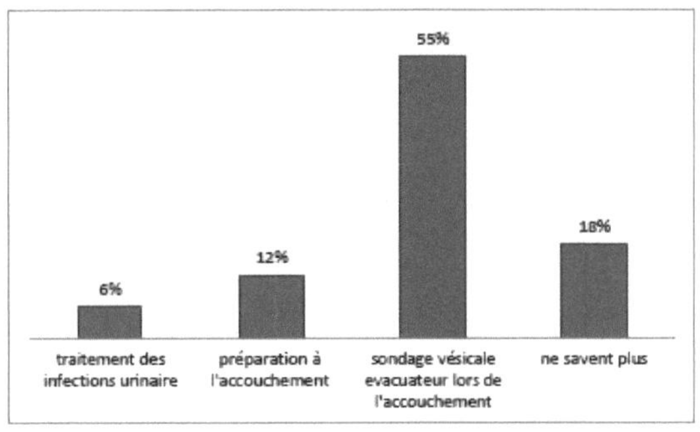

Figure 29: Preventive measures.

8. Knowledge of the treatment of urinary incontinence :

√ 70% of midwives were no longer familiar with treatments for urinary incontinence, while only 30% were familiar with treatments The midwives who answered the questions worked in different positions (Figure 30).

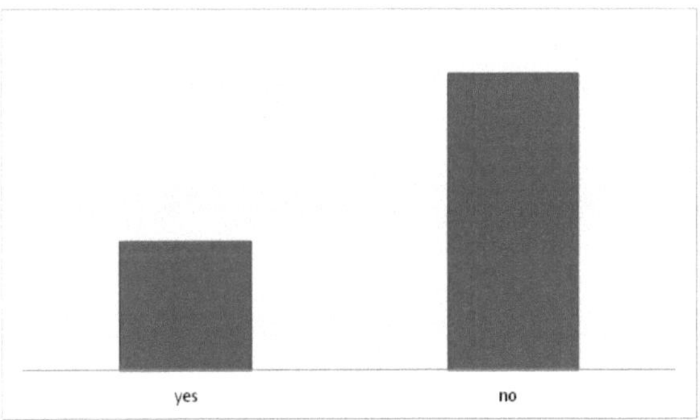

Figure 30: Distribution according to knowledge of incontinence treatment.

III. Knowledge of perineal rehabilitation :

✓ 52% of participants in the study had undergone perineal rehabilitation (Figure
31).

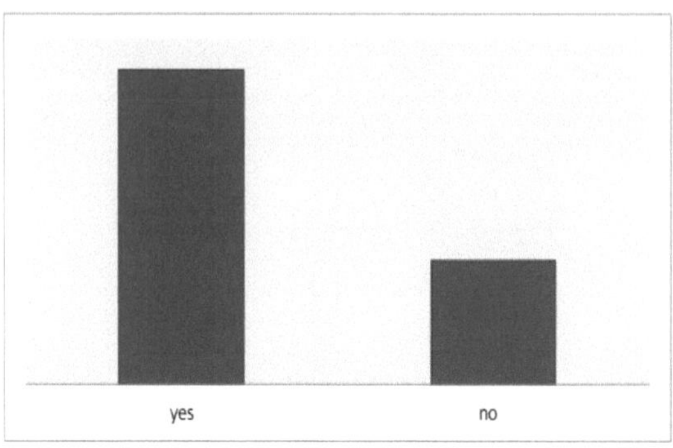

Figure 31: Knowledge of perineal rehabilitation.

1. Can you do perineal rehabilitation?

✓ 24% of midwives familiar with perineal reeducation were able to practise
perineal reeducation (Figure 32).

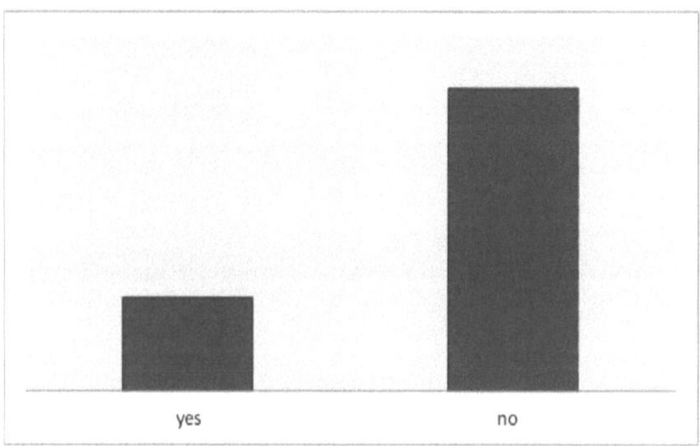

Figure 32: Knowledge of perineal rehabilitation practice.

2. Do you prescribe or recommend perineal rehabilitation?

✓ 59% of midwives who were familiar with perineal rehabilitation advised

women to undergo perineal rehabilitation sessions (Figure 33).

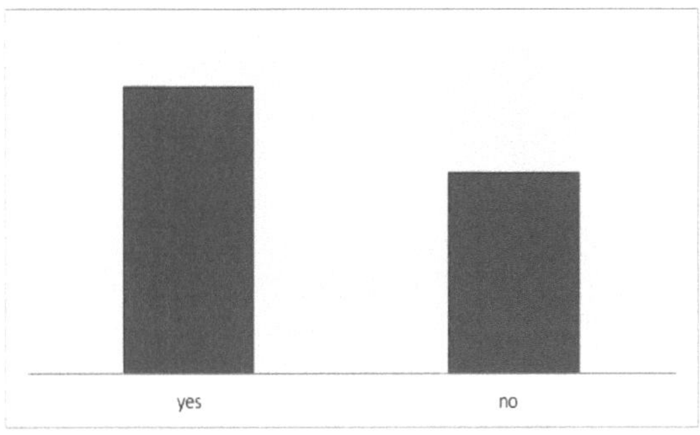

Figure 33: Prescription for perineal rehabilitation.

3. The target population :

✓ The most recommended target population was women with risk factors

(70%) (Figure 34).

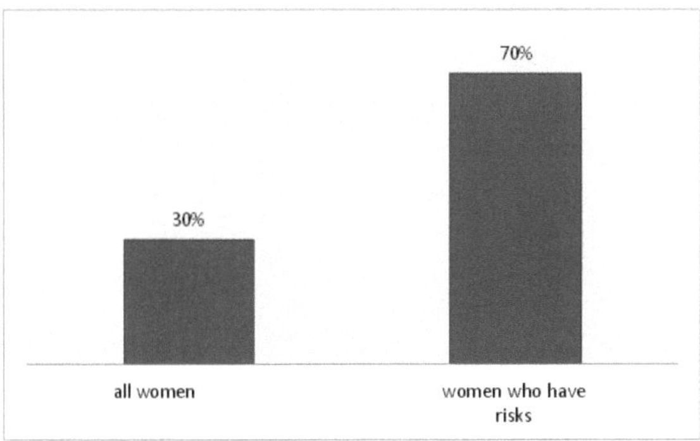

Figure 34: The population referred for perineal rehabilitation

4. Should perineal re-education be included in midwife training?

✓ All the midwives who responded to the questionnaires said that perineal rehabilitation should be included in midwifery training (Figure 35).

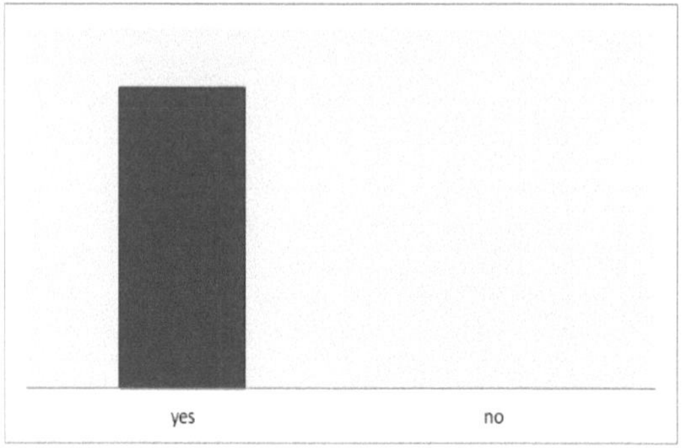

Figure 35: The desire to include perineal rehabilitation in the initial training of midwives.

5. Would you like to take a course in perineal rehabilitation?

✓ The 33 midwives who responded to the questionnaires wanted to receive training in perineal rehabilitation (figure 36).

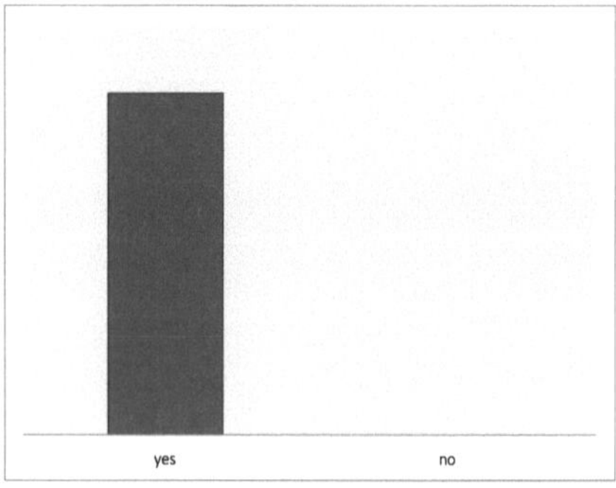

Figure 36: Desire to follow perineal rehabilitation training.

Results comparison tables

List of abbreviations :

- I^+ : number of women with postpartum urinary incontinence

- I^- : number of women who did not experience post-partum incontinence.

- NS: not significant

- S: significant

I. Parity

Incontinence parity	I+	I-	meaning
primiparous	4	24	NS
Second pare	4	21	
Third pare	5	12	

$$X^2=1.77$$

I. Weight gain

Incontinence weight gain	I+	I-	meaning
<10 kg	6	33	NS
between 10 and 15 kg	3	18	
>15 kg	2	8	

$$X^2=0.175$$

II. Urinary leakage during pregnancy

Incontinence Leak during pregnancy	I +	I-	meaning
yes	11	33	S
no	2	24	

$$X^2=4.023$$

III. Birth preparation

Incontinence preparation	I+	I-	meaning
yes	2	10	NS
no	11	47	

$$X^2=0.034$$

IV. Delivery method

incontinence mode delivery	I+	I-	meaning
AVB	9	33	NS
Forceps	1	6	
urgent c/s	2	12	
c/s programmed	1	6	

$$X^2=0.567$$

V. Lesions of the perineum

Incontinence lesions	I+	I-	meaning
no	4	17	
Simple tears	1	1	NS
Complete tears	0	0	
episiotomy	8	39	

$$X^2=1.386$$

VI. Urinary evacuation catheterisation

Incontinence catheterisation	I+	I-	meaning
yes	9	36	NS
no	4	21	

$$X^2=0.169$$

VII. Abdominal expressions

Incontinence expressions	I+	I-	meaning
yes	6	28	NS
no	7	29	

$$X^2=0.038$$

VIII. Newborn weight

Incontinence weight	I+	I-	meaning
<3.7 kg	12	45	NS
>3.7 kg	1	12	

$$X^2=1.969$$

DISCUSSION

I. Epidemiological study :

Profile of the population studied :

Half of the patients were aged between 20 and 30, as is the case in the literature [1]. 70% of patients were housewives and 40% had secondary education.

II. Background study :

1. Breakdown by parity :

The risk of a perineal tear is greater during the first vaginal delivery. This is because the perineum as a whole has never had to undergo such significant distension before. The muscles have never been stretched and are therefore more fragile during the passage of foetal presentation. However, multiparity is a risk factor for perineo-sphincter disorders. The rate of urinary incontinence is stable with parity. [2] Of the 70 patients in our study, 28 were primiparous and 42 were multiparous (36% were second parous and 24% were third parous or more). However, in our study parity had no significant influence on the occurrence of postpartum urinary incontinence.

2. Pregnancy:

a. Weight gain during pregnancy :

Normal weight gain during pregnancy is around 9 to 10 kg. Excessive weight gain is a risk factor for foetal macrosomia and more extensive tearing of the perineum. It is also an indirect risk factor for post-partum urinary incontinence. [2] In our series, half of the patients gained more than 10 kg.

b. Urinary leakage during pregnancy :

More than half of the women in our series (63%) experienced urinary leakage during pregnancy, the majority of which was cough-induced leakage (48%), a quarter was leakage with physical effort and a quarter was leakage without any effort. In the literature, one study showed an increase in the prevalence of urinary incontinence during pregnancy, with up to 32% of parturients having problems with urinary incontinence by the end of pregnancy (ref.2). Other studies have found a frequency of urinary incontinence during pregnancy of between 30% and 50% (refs. 3 and 4). Some studies even show that urinary incontinence during pregnancy is the main risk factor for post-partum urinary incontinence; in one study, 51.7% of post-partum urinary incontinence was explained by incontinence during pregnancy. In our series, urinary incontinence during pregnancy is a risk factor for the onset of urinary incontinence in the post-partum period.

c. Birth preparation :

The special case of urinary incontinence during pregnancy Perineal re-education prescribed during pregnancy as part of childbirth preparation improved urinary incontinence during pregnancy and reduced the frequency of urinary incontinence 3 months post-partum, but did not appear to have any long-term benefit. Out of 70 women, only 12 were informed and prepared for childbirth (17%). In our results, we found that preparation for birth had no influence on the onset of postpartum urinary incontinence.

III.   Study of childbirth :

1. Mode and term of delivery :

The risk of urinary incontinence was correlated with the notion of perineal trauma during pregnancy and vaginal delivery. Post-partum urinary incontinence mainly affects women who have had vaginal deliveries, although the problem also affects women who have had caesarean sections. The majority of births take place after 37 weeks of amenorrhoea Of the patients surveyed, 21 had given birth by caesarean section, 14 by emergency caesarean section and 7 by scheduled caesarean section. Of the 49 vaginal deliveries, 7 required the use of forceps. In our series, mode of delivery is not considered to be a risk factor for postpartum urinary incontinence.

2. Evacuating urinary catheter :

It is advisable to perform an evacuating bladder catheterisation before pushing. Pushing on a full bladder can cause damage to the bladder. In our study we noted that in more than half of deliveries (64%) evacuating bladder catheterisation was performed. We found that the practice of evacuating bladder catheterisation had no relationship with the onset of postpartum urinary incontinence.

3. Abdominal expression during childbirth :

During childbirth, to help with the release of the baby, very strong pressure may be exerted on the abdomen. This pressure can have serious consequences for the perineum, which is also subject to hyperpressure, and can damage muscles. In January 2007, the French National Authority for Health published the following recommendations: "There are no medically validated indications for abdominal expression". In half of the deliveries in our study, abdominal expression was performed in 49% of cases, but the results obtained show that there is no link between abdominal expression and post-partum urinary incontinence.

4. Lesions of the perineum :

30% of patients had no damage to the perineum, 3% had a simple tear, no patient had a complete tear and 67% had an episiotomy. Recourse to episiotomy is of no importance in the prevention of post-partum urinary incontinence.

5. Newborn weight :

The risks of foetal macrosomia must be identified. Fetal macrosomia increases the risk of neurological damage to the perineum. The risks of perineal lesions are increased when the cranial perimeter is greater than 35.5cm, the diameter Biparietal greater than 99mm, birth weight greater than 3700g (Ref. 5, 6). In our study we found that 81% of newborns had a birth weight of less than 3.7 kg. According to the summary table, the excess weight of the newborn did not influence the appearance of post-partum urinary incontinence.

6. Concept of perineal rehabilitation :

To the question: can you explain what perineal re-education is and what its benefits are? 4% of patients can explain in a few words what the benefits of perineal re-education are, 7% of patients have already heard of it but have no precise idea of the benefits. 89% of patients know nothing about perineal re-education. During the maternity discharge visit, in particular, it seems essential to inform maternity patients about the spontaneous evolution of perineal deficiencies and to ensure that they are aware of any perineal damage. The need to attend the post-natal consultation should also be stressed. It is during the consultation on the $40^{\text{ème}}$ day that the indication for rehabilitation treatment will be considered. The prescription for post-partum rehabilitation sessions is based on the symptoms described by the patient or detected during the clinical examination carried out during the postnatal consultation by the midwife or the gynaecologist-obstetrician (6 to 8 weeks after the birth). The only means of information was the Internet.

IV. Incontinence in the post-partum period (one month after giving birth) :

Depending on the author, post-partum urinary incontinence occurs in 15 to 50% of cases, of which 30% will heal spontaneously in 12 to 18 months and 10% will remain disabling. [3] Urinary incontinence is defined as the loss of urine without being able to stop it. hold back voluntarily. During pregnancy, most low urinary symptoms are the result of physiological changes. These symptoms may disappear or persist following alterations in labour and/or delivery. Among the 19% of patients who had incontinence problems in the postpartum period 69% were affected by urinary incontinence due to coughing, 16% by leakage. urinary leaks with physical effort and 15% with urinary leaks without physical effort.

► Plan to undergo perineal rehabilitation:

Of the 19% of patients who responded to the second questionnaire, 54% wanted to undergo perineal re-education sessions, while 46% did not find it necessary. In the literature, there are no studies carried out in Tunisia on compliance with the prescription for perineal re-education.

V. Assessment of knowledge of midwives à about urinary incontinence :

We began our survey of midwives by asking about the definition of urinary incontinence: we found that midwives' level of knowledge was satisfactory in 79% of cases. This implies that midwives are capable of providing informed education on this subject. Our series shows that 46% of midwives are aware of the different types of urinary incontinence and that the majority (73%) are able to screen for this condition. 11% of midwives confirm that screening is carried out by questioning and clinical examination [4]. 42% of midwives said that women should be screened systematically for urinary incontinence. Systematic screening for urinary incontinence is one of the five proposals for better management of post-partum urinary incontinence [4].

Only 9% know that the most ideal time to screen for post-partum urinary incontinence is from 8 weeks post-partum (Ref 8). The postnatal consultation takes place during the second month. It includes a gynaecological examination to check - that the reproductive system has returned to normal.

- look for stress urinary and anal incontinence and assess the quality of the levator muscles

Midwives have more or less important ideas about measures to prevent urinary incontinence:

- 55% used bladder evacuation during childbirth.

-12% believe that childbirth preparation can prevent urinary incontinence. [4]

-6% say that treating urinary incontinence during pregnancy is very important in preventing urinary incontinence.

Only 30% of midwives confirm that they know how to treat urinary incontinence. Regarding the treatment of post-partum urinary incontinence, 60% of midwives confirm that perineal re-education is a treatment for this type of pathology. [5]

VI. Assessment of midwives' knowledge of perineal rehabilitation

76% of midwives are not qualified to carry out perineal re-education on a practical level 59% of midwives advised perineal re-education, especially for women with risk factors (70%). Midwives are not satisfied with their training in gynaecological urology. That's why they say that re-education should be included in midwifery training and that midwives need ongoing training in women's gynaecological urology, especially in post-partum urinary incontinence and perineal re-education.

VIII. Study review :

1. The positives

The study carried out for this dissertation has the advantage of covering many points relating to perineal rehabilitation and of having precise answers to each question. This was made possible by going to each patient for the first questionnaire, in order to be able to explain the more technical questions. The sample is varied.

2. Negative points:

The study carried out for this thesis inevitably includes a number of biases. The first is the number of patients interviewed; for more accurate statistics, a larger number of patients would have had to be studied, which was impossible in the time available for this thesis. Secondly, the number of midwives was small compared to the sample of seventy women questioned. The difference may seem significant, but it is explained by the There was also a short delay in collecting the questionnaire which meant thatthe collective responses of the midwives were less objective and reliable. Finally, the negative point of this study is the short time between the two questionnaires to see the long-term evolution of patients' urinary incontinence and the contribution of rehabilitation. It would be useful to repeat the same questionnaire at a later date with the same women in order to detect the appearance of any late complications.

CONCLUSION

Urinary continence is the result of a balance between intra-urethral and urinary pressure. bladder and urethra. The International Continence Society (ICS) defines urinary incontinence as an involuntary and disturbing loss of urine. The provision of the floor pelvic floor explains that the consequence of a or muscular trauma. We began by looking at the onset of postpartum urinary incontinence, perineal rehabilitation and the opportunities for women to talk to each other during pregnancy and the postnatal period. We then drew up and carried out 70 questionnaires with 70 women who had given birth in the post-natal care unit at AZIZA OTHMENA Hospital between 10 February 2014 and 10 March 2014, and a second questionnaire with 30 midwives in order to assess their knowledge of urinary incontinence and perineal rehabilitation. We have analysed the results of our surveys in order to highlight :

- the frequency of occurrence of post-partum urinary incontinence, which is around 19% of the study population.

- risk factors for post-partum urinary incontinence; the only factor significantly influencing the onset of post-partum urinary incontinence in our study was "the occurrence of urinary incontinence during pregnancy".

-the level of knowledge of midwives about post-partum urinary incontinence (79%) and perineal rehabilitation (24%).

Too few midwives systematically ask their patients about perineal re-education and perineo-sphincter disorders during pregnancy and in the immediate aftermath of childbirth. Out of embarrassment or modesty, patients and professionals do not discuss these subjects enough. Communication and dialogue seem difficult.

In addition, some midwives wishing to practise pelvic perineal re-education sometimes feel ill-equipped. Although initial training, spread over 3 years of study, provides theoretical knowledge of perineal re-education, it is difficult to acquire practical skills, as internships are not available in hospitals.The main problem is the lack of information available to patients. This is a problem we can remedy. The level of information on perineal re-education is lacking. It seems important that all young mothers should be made aware of the concept of perineal re-education by practitioners who take the necessary time and find the right moment to provide clear and relevant information on the subject. Midwives are primary care professionals, and are now responsible for women's reproductive health. Knowledge of the perineum and its physiology should be assessed at every consultation, with or without pelvic-perineal education sessions.

BIBLIOGRAPHY

1) LECUIVRE S. (2010), PERINEO-SPHINCTER DISORDERS AND REEDUCATION PERINEALE Prise en charge durant la grossesse et les suites de couches, obstétrique, UNIVERSITE HENRI POINCARE, NANCY École de Sages- Femmes de METZ ,80pages .

2) Vivenot,C.(2010) la rééducation périnéale du post partum : observance de la prescription mémoire : obstétrique Université Henri Ponicaré , Nancy I Ecole de sages-femmes Alberts Frunhinsholz .47 pages.

3) Guillaume.S ,Fabre.Ch ,Crètinon.S , Krbat.V ,Tayrac.S , Latour.E, Leurkowich.C, Nicot.S, Battut.A, Biladen.D, Chantemps.C, Frignet.S, Girand.V, Sachet.A, Mazolf.A, Bouvier.M Guillarme.L, Girand.V, Gaufrier.M (2014) Guide pour la pratique des sages-femmes en rééducation pelvi périnéale, Collège National des Sages- femmes(CNSF), "en France " 42 pages.

4) Aubin.I (2006) Postpartum urinary incontinence: raising the issue in the consultation following childbirth. 44 pages.

5) College national of gynaecologists obstetricians 2010 – 2011 page 21 http://umvf.univ-nantes.fr/gynecologie-et-obstetrics/teaching/item22/site/html/cours.pdf.

6) Lapitan M. Pelvic floor muscle strengthening for the prevention and treatment of urinary and faecal incontinencein women before and after childbirth: BSG Commentary (last updated: 1 April 2009). WHO Reproductive Health Library;

Geneva: World Health Organization.

7) M. ROTZETTER-OTERO (2006). HEALTH OF WOMEN 18 YEARS

AFTER AN ANAL SPHINCTER TEAR AT CHILDBIRTH: FAECAL

INCONTINENCE, URINARY INCONTINENCE AND SEXUALITY. PDF :

Department of Gynaecology-Obstetrics. Thesis presented to the Faculty of

Medicine of the University of Geneva .42pages

8) Humburg.J(2011) Urinary incontinence in women: what to do in the family

doctor's surgery page 835 pages

9) Jaquetin.B, Fauconnier.A, Fritel.X, Mellier.G, Robain.G, Haab.G, Gosson.M,

(2009), Extrait de mise à jour en gynécologie et obstétrique : Recommandation

pour la pratique clinique : Diagnostic et prise en charge de l'incontinence

urinaire de la femme adulte, Collège National des gynécologues et obstétriciens

français (CNGOF) le 17 Décembre 2009 en Paris. From page 621 to 632.

10. Neyroud, midwife, le 25 March 2014 http://www.jcomjeune.com/article-

job/midwifery

12) Mason L, Glenn S, Walton I, Appleton C. The prevalence of stress

incontinence during pregnancy and following delivery. Midwifery 1999;

15:120-128.

13) Viktrup L, Lose G, Rolff M, Barfoed K. The symptom of stress incontinence

caused by pregnancy or delivery in primiparas, Obstet Gynecol, 1992

14) Viktrup L, Lose G, Rolff M, Barfoed K, The symptom of stress incontinence

caused by pregnancy or delivery in primipara, Obstet Gynecol, 1992

15) Mørkved S, Bø K, Schei B, Salvesen KA, Pelvic Floor Muscle Training During Pregnancy to PreventUrinary Incontinence: A Single-Blind Randomized Control Trial, Obstet Gynecol, 2003

16) De Leeuw, Vierhout, Struijk, Hop, Wallenburg, Anal sphincter damage after vaginal delivery: functional outcome and risk factors for fecal incontinence, Acta Obstetricia and Gynecologica, Scandinavica, 2001

17) Handa, Danielsen, Gilbert, Obstetric anal sphincter lacerations, Obstet Gynecol, 2001

18) JOUFFROY Bénédicte. Indication de la rééducation périnéale postnatale, 10 mai 2006, Strasbourg, pp 75-88.

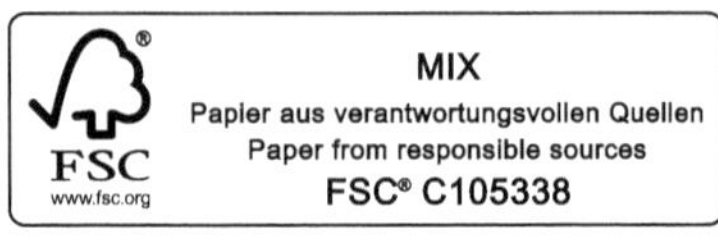

Printed by Books on Demand GmbH, Norderstedt / Germany